MW01148444

To Jo-Ann & Michael
To my dear dear friends -
With all best wishes +
much, much love,

Sunny Buchman

Jo-Ann, my soul mate -
How can I ever thank you
enough Jo-Ann, for all
you did to help make this
book come to fruition,
Thank you, especially for
all the support you've
given me since I've
met you.

Precious Window of Time

"This book is as beautiful as it is filled with wisdom. If someone you love has dementia, this book will enhance both of your lives."

—Stacey Mandelbaum, MD

This is an enlightened description of the life of a husband with Alzheimer's disease and his loving caregiver wife. It is unique in that it is told from the viewpoint of both the patient and his wife in a series of interviews she conducted and recorded. The practical and spiritual approach used here turns this possibly distressful tale into a model for caregivers.

—Orel Friedman, MD, gerontologist (retired)

This extraordinarily insightful, personal, and practical book is a must-read for anyone wanting to help a person with Alzheimer's function at their personal best, at each progressive stage of this disease.

—Jo-Ann Friedman Rapaport
Author of *Home Health Care:
A Complete Guide for Patients and Their Families*

During my thirty-year nursing career, I have witnessed the devastation that Alzheimer's disease can leave in its terrible wake. Sunny and Paul refused to let this awful disease take control. Their amazing story is one of honest transparency, a truly inspiring account of their journey of unconditional love filled with dignity, courage, and a promise to live each moment to the fullest. Imagine what a different place our world would be if we all practiced the "ing" philosophy described within these pages. I hope that the reader, whether a person stricken by this disease or a loved one trying to cope with Alzheimer's, will gain invaluable insight on how to maintain a meaningful quality of life and will realize how to make each moment count as the Buchmans have done so successfully. Kudos to Sunny and Paul for serving as such an inspiring example for us all!

—Tammy Hunter-Heckenberg
Adirondack Alzheimer's Advisory Council

Precious Window of Time

OUR JOURNEY WITH ALZHEIMER'S DISEASE

Sunny Buchman with Paul Buchman

authorHOUSE®

AuthorHouse™
1663 Liberty Drive
Bloomington, IN 47403
www.authorhouse.com
Phone: 1-800-839-8640

© *2011 Sunny Buchman with Paul Buchman. All rights reserved.*

No part of this book may be reproduced, stored in a retrieval system, or transmitted by any means without the written permission of the author.

First published by AuthorHouse 10/4/2011

ISBN: 978-1-4670-3770-9 (e)
ISBN: 978-1-4670-3771-6 (sc)

Library of Congress Control Number: 2011916941

Printed in the United States of America

Any people depicted in stock imagery provided by Thinkstock are models, and such images are being used for illustrative purposes only. Certain stock imagery © *Thinkstock.*

This book is printed on acid-free paper.

Because of the dynamic nature of the Internet, any web addresses or links contained in this book may have changed since publication and may no longer be valid. The views expressed in this work are solely those of the author and do not necessarily reflect the views of the publisher, and the publisher hereby disclaims any responsibility for them.

DEDICATION

*T*his book is dedicated to my beloved husband, Paul, and would not have been possible without his willingness.

It is also dedicated to our children and their spouses—Rebecca, Rachel and Mark, and Joshua and Carol—and their children Noa, Mika, Eden, Jessica, Jason, Danielle, Tyler, Kalie, and Talia. Their support and love carry us through each day.

Finally, I wish to dedicate this book to both of our beloved mothers, Clara Yanklowitz Aronson and Dorothy Friedland Buchman, who suffered from Alzheimer's disease.

CONTENTS

ACKNOWLEDGMENTS

My special thanks to Chandler Atkins, my psychology professor, who many years ago encouraged me to write a book about the aging process. I am grateful to him for his belief in me.

I am indebted to Rebecca Kimelman, Rachel Lipschutz, Joshua Buchman, Michele Gottlieb, Stacey Mandelbaum, Jo-Ann Friedman Rapaport, Bill Everett, Joan Robertson, Stacey Morris, Sharon Bogdan, Rena Bernstein, Vlad Morozov, Sujata Chaudhry, Helen Cackener, Karen Northrup, Jane Canaday Hawn, Mimi and Howard Hirsch, Barbara and Barry Ziff, Irene Buchman, Sarah O'Higgins, Cory Seelye Dixon, Joan and By Lapham, and Mel Krug for their help, inspiration, guidance, and encouragement.

Thanks, also, to our many family members and friends, too numerous to name, who read the book in its manuscript form and gave me input and helpful feedback.

I am deeply grateful to the following physicians for helping Paul: Dr. Richard P. Leach Jr., internist; Dr. Ronald Stram of the Center for Integrative Health and Healing; Dr.

Samuel Gottesman, urologist; Dr. Jonathan M. DeSantis, cardiologist; and Dr. Richard Holub, neurologist.

The Glen at Hiland Meadows, Queensbury, New York—the independent living facility we moved to six years ago—has been a blessing. Words cannot describe how grateful I am to the staff and residents of The Glen. The staff has gone above and beyond the call of duty to meet our needs, and the residents have offered unconditional friendship and support.

Proceeds from each book sold will be donated to the Alzheimer's Association of Northeastern New York to benefit programs and services in the Adirondack region.

Chapter 1
THEN AND NOW

*I*n the years before Paul's Alzheimer's diagnosis, he was a self-employed wholesale food distributor; he was most proud of having been the first-ever distributor of Ben & Jerry's ice cream. In addition to his vocation, his passions included opera, ballet, music, and (watching) all sports, especially the Yankees. He was a lifelong learner, and after retiring, he audited courses at the local college regularly. Paul read voraciously. He was a people person. He had an even disposition and everyone loved him. He made no waves. He worked long hours at Eastern Food Supply, his food service business. He served on many boards, including the Crandall Public Library, the World Awareness Children's Museum, and Synagogue Congregation Shaaray Tefila, and he was president of the Lake George Opera Festival. Paul was a highly respected member of the community.

Several years ago, Paul and I went to the Lahey Clinic near Boston for Paul to have a complete physical exam. Paul wasn't doing well, and although I couldn't articulate what was happening, he wasn't "Paul." He had been going to a range of specialists, but an overview was needed.

We came away devastated. The doctors discovered that Paul's arteries were clogged once again, even though he had had a quadruple heart bypass operation years before. He was also told that he needed a prostate operation, that he had stenosis of the back for which he should see a surgeon, and that he should also see a neurologist. The recommendation for Paul to see a neurologist came as a complete surprise. I was so focused on the physical aspects of Paul's health that I hadn't paid enough attention to the strange behaviors he was exhibiting. For instance, I didn't catch that a significant change in how Paul was recording his business transactions had taken place. Or that his judgment was not solid—for example, he would cross a street without first checking for oncoming traffic.

Lahey Clinic made the appointment with the neurologist for that same day, and this doctor told us that Paul had Alzheimer's disease. As you can imagine, both Paul and I were shocked, and we left depressed and utterly discouraged.

We came home and tackled one problem after another. I sought the best doctors I could find in the Glens Falls-Albany and surrounding area and showed them the findings from the Lahey Clinic. The local urologist performed Paul's prostate operation. A decision was made to hold off on performing surgery on Paul's back.

Concurrently, I took Paul to a holistic doctor who

put him on supplements to replace medication wherever possible and encouraged him to improve his eating habits by keeping a chart of his food intake and drinking nourishing smoothies. He motivated Paul to begin an exercise regimen and put Paul on an antidepressant. Paul responded to this new approach, and even though he was confused at times, he came back to the living.

Reaching agreement regarding the diagnosis of Alzheimer's disease, however, was not an easy process. Fortunately or unfortunately, in spite of the initial diagnosis made by the neurologist at the Lahey Clinic, Paul passed the diagnostic tests administered by local doctors with flying colors. Since Paul majored in math and English in college, these sections of the tests were very easy for him.

Finally, four neurologists later, a proper diagnosis was made and was accompanied by a plausible explanation. The doctor stated, "Paul, these tests work well for almost everyone, but *you* fall between the cracks." I later learned that this can happen to patients with above-average intelligence. And while this is not typical, in Paul's case, his high level of performance on the tests reflected his native intelligence, masking his condition of deterioration. Paul was put on Aricept; at a later date, Namenda was added.

Paul experienced the phases that most people go through with Alzheimer's disease—denial, frustration, anger, agitation, confusion, roaming or wandering, loss of memory, loss of reasoning, loss of judgment, and the inability to make choices. His personality changed as well. He became very argumentative.

Throughout this time, I too was frustrated, angry, confused, and often at my wits' end. Life became so difficult and stressful that I would pray each night that I would be able to make it through the next day. Paul would go off skiing by himself, and I would worry that he could ski safely and find his way home. He loved to do our grocery shopping, but he would often bring back the opposite of what I had requested. Even when I insisted he take a shopping list, he might forget to look at it or even remember he had a list with him. As he left the house, if I said, "Paul, we need sweet potatoes," he would come home with white potatoes. I bought cell phones to help, but Paul would forget to take his, or he would forget where it was or how to use it.

I couldn't figure out what was happening, and I had conflicting feelings. Was he intentionally doing this to get me upset? I wasn't sure if this was passive aggression—his way of showing anger—or if something else was going on. Eventually, I recognized that he wasn't deliberately trying to upset me, but rather, he lacked the understanding that he could no longer remember. This insight allowed me to shed my anger and deal with what was causing the problem: the Alzheimer's.

When the diagnosis was confirmed, I sought help from a therapist. I found myself crying and using up boxes of his tissues in one sitting. I was stuck in my grief. I wanted to scream! I was grieving the death of our marriage as I knew it, the slow death of the person I loved, and the sadness of knowing our lives were forever changed. However, I knew it was necessary to go through the grieving stage first before acceptance could take place, and I was grateful for help in my grieving. I realized it was essential to seek professional help. I needed this help in order to move forward.

Wisely, I came to the conclusion that whatever number of years Paul and I had left, we would live them in a positive way. I was determined to eliminate any unnecessary stress and devote my energies to our relationship. First, I made the crucial decision to move. Despite the fact that our home of over thirty-five years was important to our family, with many beautiful memories, I knew it was time to simplify our life. We sold our house and moved to The Glen at Hiland Meadows, a senior independent-living community. Not long after we moved, The Glen offered a free six-week program for caregivers of Alzheimer's patients. That program was called "The Savvy Caregiver," and it gave me tools that I then creatively adapted and used to turn our lives from despair to coping and finally to great happiness. I also began attending the once-a-month Alzheimer's support group and began reading everything I could about Alzheimer's disease.

I learned that every person's journey with the disease will be different, but there are tools that will be helpful for everyone. For the past few years, friends have urged me to write this book. They wanted people to be able to gain ideas from our experience. I hope our thoughts, words, and suggestions prove to be a guide and inspiration for others. This book is about facing the realities of Alzheimer's with a focus on seeing the positive side of the disease. Yes, there is a positive side!

Without question, living with Alzheimer's is terrible. Alzheimer's is an insidious disease. Currently, there is no cure; there is only the buying of time. But my purpose in writing this book is to show how precious that window of time is, and that it can be a very special time for both the person with Alzheimer's and for the caregiver. I know for us, the other shoe will drop before too long, but I intend to make the most of these years before it does.

At this point in the disease, Paul has no memory of being told by several doctors that he has Alzheimer's disease. Recently, when I asked him if he remembers the workup tests or the MRI that helped determine that he had Alzheimer's, he said no.

During the test at each visit to the neurologist, Paul can no longer retain the three words he is given and then later asked to recall. He says he doesn't mind being tested. He tries hard to answer the questions. Paul's short-term memory is all but gone. His long-term memory is also on the decline, as is his ability to process.

Incredibly, even today, many people are unaware that Paul has Alzheimer's, as he is able to compensate so well. Socially, Paul has always been gifted, and this serves him especially well now. He appears normal and knows how to steer a conversation by asking questions. As a result, people aren't realizing that they are doing most of the talking, not Paul. Another way Paul has compensated is by writing crib notes. For example, before getting together with other people, Paul will write their names on a scrap of paper, stick it in his pocket, and practice them several times.

On January 26, 2010, we celebrated our fifty-second wedding anniversary. Paul gave me the best anniversary present ever. Just before bedtime, he suddenly turned to me and said, "I must say, Sunny, that every day I thank your mother and father for giving birth to you!"

Like most couples, we have had ups and downs in our married life, but our shared values, our shared interests, and most importantly, our deep love for each other have helped give us the determination to make a success of our marriage. We have three remarkable children (and their special spouses) and nine wonderful grandchildren. In spite of the great geographic distances that separate us, we are a very close and loving family. We are truly blessed.

Chapter 2
A Positive Approach to Alzheimer's: The "Ings" Interview

*A*t this midpoint in the disease, Paul is unable to carry on a deep conversation with anyone. He never was comfortable expressing how he felt. As his caregiver, though, I was anxious to know what he was thinking and feeling.

I devised a plan. By creating questions and interviewing Paul, I hoped to help him share his thoughts and feelings with me. Through this, I would try to find the way to best help him and keep the windows of our lives propped open.

Together, we thought of and listed words that end in "ing." As the interviewer, I would first ask Paul his thoughts, and I would then couple his response with my feelings and perspective as his caregiver. I've called my part of these "Sunny's Reflection."

I gained Paul's cooperation by presenting the interview as an activity we could do together. Since so much of what we had previously participated in as a couple was no longer possible, this shared effort was a real bonus.

Although at this point in time Paul was already having difficulty with anything other than superficial conversation, I found that if I asked him only one question a day, he would, with great effort, be able to answer. It wasn't easy for him to process the questions, and he was exhausted after each session. Because of his Alzheimer's, he often gave short answers. However, as I had hoped, his responses to the following words ending in "ing" provided a window that gave me excellent insight into his thoughts and feelings.

By focusing on the positive "ings"—such as loving, hugging, touching, laughing, accepting—I have been able to turn what could easily have been the worst years of our lives into the best years of our lives. The changes brought about by Alzheimer's disease can be devastating, or they can present an opportunity to grow even closer together. As we concentrate on the "ings," Paul's and my love for each other has deepened. Every day presents an opportunity, and the "ings" in life have helped provide me with the tools.

What follows is my interview with Paul, including my reflections and insights on each "ing."

Loving

Sunny: How important is loving to you?

Paul: *Very! In capital letters!* More than ever before, I love my wife. Loving my family is very important. But I say "I like" friends, not "I love" them.

Sunny: How important is it for other people loving you?

Paul: That's important also. I don't want to be isolated in the world. I feel my wife loves me very much. I can feel her love, and I need it. It's crucial for me. Also, the love and respect of my children, grandchildren, and friends help me feel good about myself. I have a lot of love to give, and I appreciate and am grateful for the love shown me.

Sunny's Reflection: I love Paul with all my heart, and I know that my loving Paul unconditionally is critical. Even when the disease makes him do things that are not lovable, I focus on being loving. I know that it is the disease that causes him to act in unacceptable ways. I mentally put my heart inside his heart. As Paul so eloquently expressed, the feeling of being loved is incredibly important to the Alzheimer's patient.

Hugging

Sunny: Do you like hugging? Is it a good feeling?
Paul: *Yes!* And *yes!*

Sunny: Is hugging important?

11

Paul: Absolutely!

Sunny's Reflection: We try to hug many times throughout the day. With a good hug, words aren't needed. So much comfort can be conveyed through a hug. Both the giver and the receiver benefit—Paul's hugs help me, and my hugs help him. People often ask Paul if he would give them a hug. People all the time say, "Paul, you're the best hugger!"

Touching

Sunny: Do you like when I touch you?
Paul: *Yes! Very much!*

Sunny: Do you think touching is important for you?
Paul: The feeling of touching is an important one—shaking hands, hugging, kissing, etc.

Sunny: Has touching always been important to you or more so in the last few years?
Paul: It has always been important to me.

Sunny's Reflection: I'm aware of how important touching is to Paul, and I touch him as often as possible. I touch him often so that he actually feels my love for him even when he has difficulty processing words. Also, I need his touching as much as he needs mine. At night, in bed, reaching out with my toes and touching his is such a reassuring feeling for me. It reminds me of how fortunate we are that we are still together.

Laughing

Sunny: Is laughing important?

Paul: Yes, it's extremely important. I get a chance to laugh. I'm very lucky. I'm still able to make jokes. I'm not a joke teller any more, but I still have a good sense of humor, and I love to make people laugh. People should be able to laugh at themselves. Example: "Oh, you bowled 252, Sunny! I did too, only it was 126 and 126!"

Sunny's Reflection: Paul loves to be amusing. He can still make jokes. It definitely helps and is essential for the caregiver, also, to keep a sense of humor. Paul makes me smile often. When I had to call the hospital to preregister him for a colonoscopy and needed his Medicare card, I asked him, "Is your wallet around?" and he quickly replied, "No, it's square." Whenever Paul holds the door for someone, he will jokingly say, "I work on tips, you know." And then he will add, "You're supposed to say number four in the seventh race." And when someone calls on the phone, he will say, "Usually there is an extra charge to talk to me, but because it's you, there's no charge."

Crying

Sunny: Paul, do you ever cry about having Alzheimer's?

Paul: I never even think about it.

Sunny's Reflection: I don't know what Paul understands about having Alzheimer's. I sense that in the beginning, he was aware that he had memory loss. As time has passed, I don't believe he realizes he has Alzheimer's disease, because he is unable to process information related to his medical condition. His response, "I never even think about it," most likely reflects his inability to process this reality rather than a loss of emotional ability.

Accepting

Sunny: Paul, do you know what *Alzheimer's* means?

Paul: Yes, I accept it. It's not scary. I'm just accepting it.

Sunny's Reflection: Actually, Paul doesn't remember what it means. Just before I asked him this question, he asked me what *Alzheimer's* meant, and I told him it meant memory loss. Paul doesn't remember that he has Alzheimer's. When I explained it to him, he said, "More and more, I'm realizing that I have a lack of memory. I know I have to ask you what day of the week it is and the date two or three times a day. Also, I've told you to please not ask me to do more than one thing at a time." He is very aware that he can only handle one task at a time. In general, however, he seems oblivious to the fact that he has Alzheimer's. I know he can't remember the doctor explaining that he has Alzheimer's.

Worrying

Sunny: Do you ever find yourself worrying?

Paul: I don't worry. I know I can always look it up in the dictionary.

Sunny's Reflection: It seems as though Paul no longer possesses the ability to worry about practical matters. I worry for the both of us about the future. I also worry if I am up to the task of caregiving, and I worry if I will be able to keep Paul here with me. Every day presents new challenges. But I realize the importance of living in the now and taking one day at a time. I look forward to each day and rejoice in the new day as an opportunity to learn and to grow. Every day presents challenges, while at the same time presenting me with ways to grow. I have learned to channel my worries, and I've presented these strategies in Chapter 6 of this book.

Challenging

Sunny: What are you finding to be your biggest challenges?

Paul: To remember names. My lack of interest to read a book. Remembering appointments. Staying alert—I feel like sleeping all the time. Frustration at not being allowed to drive. Math is still no problem. Reading the words is no problem. However, reading a book is a problem. I can't remember what goes before. I am aware that I don't participate in conversations as much as I did. Walking is a challenge because of my back. I don't exercise as much as I used to, but I'm aware that I should.

Sunny's Reflection: One of Paul's biggest challenges has been allowing me to help him, especially with his medicines. One of my challenges was taking charge of everything. It was overwhelming at first. Paul had always taken care of our finances, and suddenly without preparation I was responsible for everything, including all decisions. One of the most challenging times was when the doctor informed him he was not to drive anymore. He went ballistic. He was determined he would still drive and was miserable in every sense of the word. I made him give me his set of keys, and that infuriated him. He kept insisting that he was a better driver than I was, and I assured him that was probably true. Taking away his driving was one of the hardest hurdles to overcome. I remained calm but firm, and he finally, sadly, accepted that his driving days were over. Fortunately, I am not afraid of challenges and meet them head on. More on facing challenges can be found in the last section of this book.

Asking (Over and Over)

Sunny: Are you aware that you are asking me questions all day long?

Paul: I'm aware that every morning I ask you, "Do we have anything on the calendar for today?" And that I have to continually ask you people's names. I know I have to ask you more and more questions as time goes by. I feel free to ask you. You don't seem to mind.

Sunny's Reflection: Paul is not aware that he continually asks me the same questions over and over again many times. Sometimes it is hard for me not to lose it! It can really wear me out to have him keep asking the same question every few seconds, but it is teaching me patience and understanding. Remembering people's names presents a major problem for Paul, but I keep assuring him that I am there to be his memory, and that I don't mind him asking me. To help him, I encourage him to write things down instead of relying on memory. Mostly he insists he doesn't need to write it down, that he will remember, which of course he can't. Whenever I leave the apartment, I write a note to tell Paul where I am going to be, and I leave the note in the same place on the table each time. I've trained him to do the same.

Supporting

Sunny: Are there people who are supportive of you?
Paul: Yes! Family and friends.

Sunny: Is it important?
Paul: I think so.

Sunny: In what way can they be supportive?
Paul: They try to cheer me up when I'm not feeling well. To be friendly and caring and helpful is very supportive. I think networking is important for you to keep in touch with the world and not keep you isolated.

Sunny's Reflection: Both the person with Alzheimer's disease and the caregiver need support, and they need a supportive network. Our three children are our biggest source of support. Their emotional support to both Paul and me has been invaluable. We have a pact that I will be completely honest with them and not try to protect them from what is happening. They are willing to help us in any way we need help. Our siblings, too, are incredibly supportive. Especially helpful are friends who come to go for walks with me in the vicinity of The Glen. That way I get my exercise and fresh air, and I get to keep in touch with my friends. The staff at The Glen as well as the residents have been wonderfully supportive. In addition, we have great support from the Alzheimer's Association. It means a great deal to know I can call the association's helpline any time, twenty-four hours a day.

Socializing

Sunny: Is socializing important to you?

Paul: The reason I like socializing is that I look forward to learning from other people. It's nice to be with all the people at the Happy Hour at The Glen.

Sunny's Reflection: Paul has always loved socializing. He is a "people person," and The Glen is ideal for him. He can always find someone around to talk with. Paul was an outstanding conversationalist; however, it is growing harder and harder for him to process meaningful conversations. He is much quieter now when he goes to Happy Hour, and he listens more than he speaks. He is still excellent at superficial chatting. Mainly, Paul asks everyone the same questions: "Did you get to play your eighteen holes of golf today?" or "Do you have any travel plans for the winter?" Also, he relies on set stories for his conversations. He often relates that he was co-author of the sports page of his college newspaper with Harvey Milk, or how his birth changed the course of history (he was born on the eve of the Great Depression of 1929).

Helping

Sunny: What does helping mean to you? How do you feel about helping? Is it important to you to still be able to help? In what ways do you help?

Paul: It's important in getting along with others in life. It makes good friends, good neighbors, good family. It gives me a good feeling to help others. I straighten the bed in the morning, I do the dishes. I do it to relieve you. I bring the mail to the apartment. I take out the trash. I fold the laundry after it has been washed and dried. When we have company I try to be a good host. I take their coats. I help push the women's chairs into the dining-room table. When we have a program like a play, I greet people and hand out the programs.

Sunny's Reflection: One day, out of the blue, Paul started washing the dishes. I told him it wasn't necessary, but he was insistent that he wanted to do it. From then on, he would insist that he wanted to wash the dishes. It was then that I realized that he wanted to do something to be helpful. I found ways that he could help, and it increased his self-esteem. It meant a lot to him to be able to help in whatever way he could. The Alzheimer's program I attended stressed the importance of letting the patient do things like folding clothes. One night a month, I am expected to help out at our synagogue's Bingo night. I requested a certain job that had two parts and told Paul I needed his assistance to do the job of handing each player a plastic garbage bag. He said he would do it to help me. We sit at a table, and I sell the cards for two extra games, and Paul sits next to me and hands out the bags. He jokes and chats with each player. They joke and chat back. They love him. One lady rubs the top of his bald head each time for good luck! He loves helping and looks forward to our once-a-month responsibility.

Eating / Snacking

Sunny: In the last few years, have you seen any changes in your eating?

Paul: Not that I'm aware of. But I often say to you, Sunny, "The older I get, the less hungry I am." I do have a great craving for chocolate—*anything* chocolate! I was always prone to snacking. That hasn't changed. Also, I've lost my sense of taste. I have a smaller appetite at mealtimes now. I still enjoy eating!

Sunny's Reflection: Paul doesn't remember that in the morning, he will go down to the lunchroom and sit and drink coffee and eat Danish pastries for several hours as he reads the paper. Then he comes up to the apartment for lunch and tells me that he's noticing that the older he gets, he doesn't seem to be as hungry. He can't remember that he has been eating all morning while reading the paper. Or at other times, he will forget that he has had a large bowl of ice cream and will go and get another. Paul definitely still enjoys eating—especially chocolate desserts!

Sleeping

Sunny: In the last few years, have you seen any changes in your sleeping?

Paul: I sleep more. I require longer hours of sleep, and sometimes I take an afternoon nap. A possible factor may be that I have to get up at night to go to the bathroom, and therefore, I don't get a straight full night's sleep.

Sunny's Reflection: Sleeping is a major problem for Paul. It is hard for him to fall asleep at night, and he is up many times during the night. He seems to get his best sleep in the morning. He feels bad that he often requires a nap in the afternoon, but I assure him that it is a good idea for him to nap when he needs it.

Reading

Sunny: You have always been a voracious reader. Has there been any change?

Paul: Yes, I read fewer books and instead spend more time at the computer. It's harder and harder for me to read a book. Reading the daily paper is still very important to me. I understand what I'm reading, but a few minutes later I can't remember what I read.

Sunny's Reflection: Paul's reading ability is still intact, but reading a book has become too difficult for him since he has to remember the characters and plot. When asked to read aloud at our spiritual journey monthly meeting, he reads beautifully and with excellent expression. He is the best reader at the session, and he gets pleasure and kudos out of doing this. However, he can't retain what he reads.

Enjoying

Sunny: What do you enjoy most?

Paul: 1. Watching sports—live games, TV games, baseball, football, basketball, hockey. 2. Being with family. 3. Spending quiet times with my wife. 4. Going to concerts. 5. Socializing. 6. Eating anything chocolate. 7. Inviting friends to join us for dinner. 8. Doing crossword puzzles all day and night long. 9. Watching the Yankees play and especially winning the World Series!

Sunny's Reflection: I try to join Paul's world. I never was interested in baseball, but I started watching the Yankee games with him and am now hooked! I arrange for us to go to hockey games that he loves and to concerts, which we both love. We used to attend plays, but he no longer enjoys them. Whatever doesn't work anymore, I eliminate. I try to keep aware of what works and what doesn't work.

Praying

Sunny: How important do you think praying is for you?

Paul: I feel it's important when I do it, but I don't seek out times just to pray. However, I don't mind going for short religious services and especially to help make the minyan. (Ten people are required in order to say special prayers like the Kaddish, the prayer for the deceased.)

Sunny: How do you feel about praying on someone's behalf (intercessory prayer)?

Paul: It's very important, and I don't mind doing it. It's important to help others. Also, I am very grateful to God and thank God every day for my wife and the good life I have.

Sunny's Reflection: I encourage Paul to continue to sing the Kiddush, the blessing over wine, every Friday night at our Friday evening meal and to say the blessing over the bread. This helps him maintain his self-esteem. He also remembers all the melodies of the prayers we sing at services. I know it gives him a very good feeling to be able to chant the blessings and prayers. He also joins me in singing the blessings over the candles at Chanukah time.

Forgiving

Sunny: Do you have any forgiving you need to do?

Paul: Not that I can think of. I try not to postpone anything like that.

Sunny's Reflection: Paul never carries a grudge. He gets along well with everyone. It's hard to think of any time he would need to ask someone's forgiveness. On the other hand, as his caretaker, I need to forgive myself for the times I become angry, such as when he hides his dirty Depends in the closet instead of putting them in the garbage, or when I'm tired and he continually asks the same question over and over. I was extremely angry when he got away from me in Penn Station in New York City and I couldn't find him for half an hour. He had no idea why I was so upset. I always feel so bad after I have lost my temper, because I know he isn't doing these things to be mean or to get at me. I know it is the disease, and I feel so terrible each time I blow up. The good news is that he doesn't seem to remember those episodes and doesn't hold them against me. I have also had to forgive him for being sick, as I know that is not his choice. It is similar to raising a child. I need to always be on the alert for his safety and well-being.

Caregiving

Sunny: Do you have any comments about my care of you?

Paul: I'm very, very happy. I think you do a great job, Sunny!

Sunny's Reflection: The most important thing for me as Paul's caregiver is to remember that I must take care of myself. I constantly remind myself that I have to stay healthy and upbeat. Paul feeds off of me. If he sees me happy and fulfilled, he is happy. Right after we moved, I realized I looked worn out, and I decided I needed to focus on myself. I bought some new clothes, got a new hairstyle, and with all the compliments I was receiving, I felt great. This, in turn, helped Paul to feel great. Caregiving can be frustrating and exhausting, but it can also be rewarding, and it is such a good feeling to be able to help the one I love.

Growing

Sunny: Do you feel you have grown at all over the past five years?

Paul: I think I've learned from living here at The Glen and from speaking with residents how to be happier and more content. The residents have been role models for me.

Sunny's Reflection: What a beautiful response! And it's true. Paul has grown in many ways. And he is happier and more content since we are living here. The majority of the residents are in their late eighties and nineties. We have learned a great deal from them. The residents and staff are warm, loving, and supportive, and help provide a perfect atmosphere for our needs.

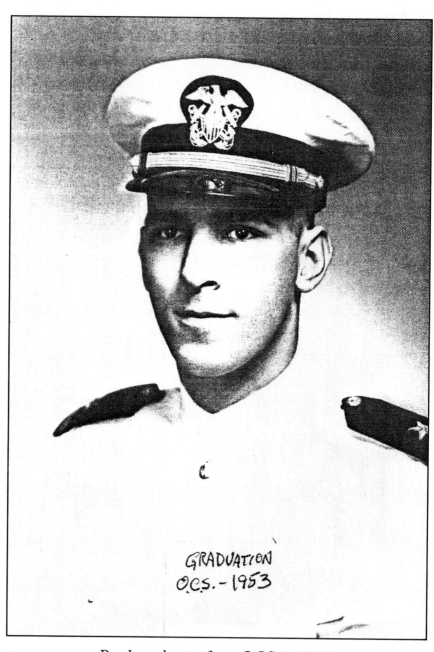

GRADUATION
O.C.S. - 1953

Paul graduates from OCS in 1953.

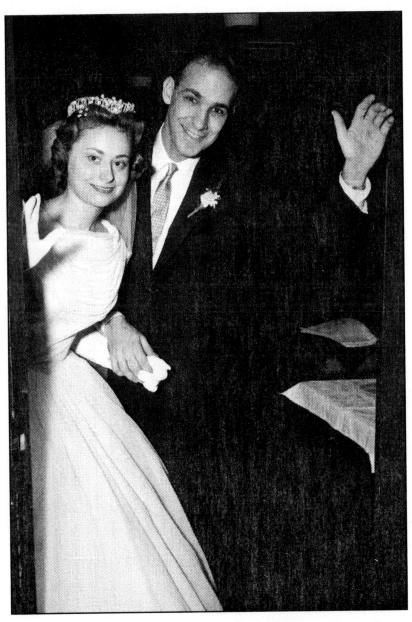

*We met in October of 1957, were engaged in December
and married on January 26, 1958. It
was a whirlwind courtship.*

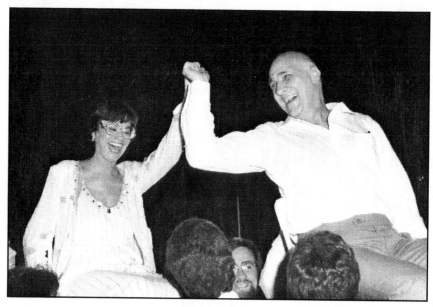

In traditional Jewish custom, as the parents of the bride, we were lifted on chairs in celebration at our daughter Rebecca's wedding in Israel in 1987.

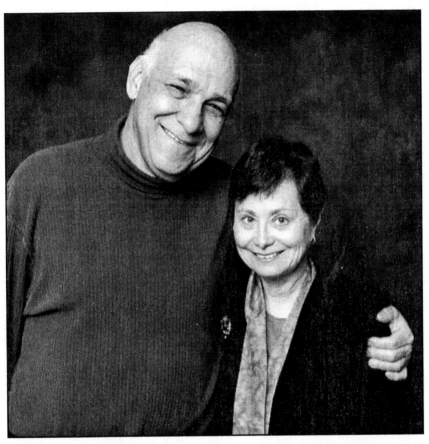

*This photo of Paul and me was taken by our good friend
Jamie Margolis during our annual visit to Israel in 2000.*

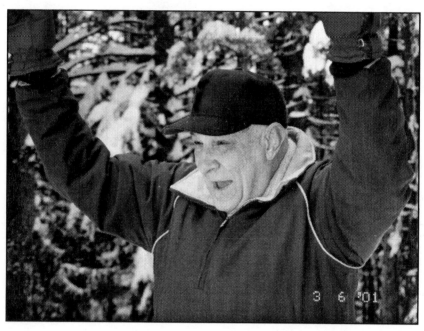

Paul loved to ski and here he is enthusiastically enjoying Spring skiing in 2001.

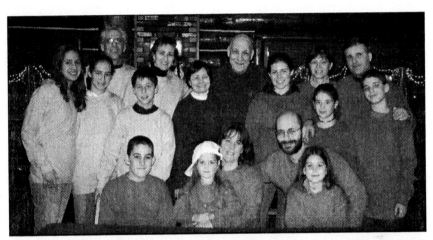

In December of 2004, our three children and their spouses and our nine grandchildren joined us for a vacation together at a ranch in Warrensburg, NY to celebrate Paul's 75th birthday.

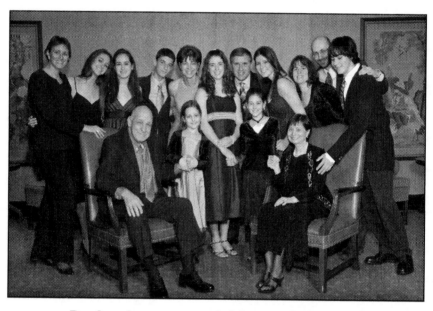

*Paul and me surrounded by our children and
grandchildren at our granddaughter Danielle
Lipschutz's Bat Mitzvah in March of 2007.*

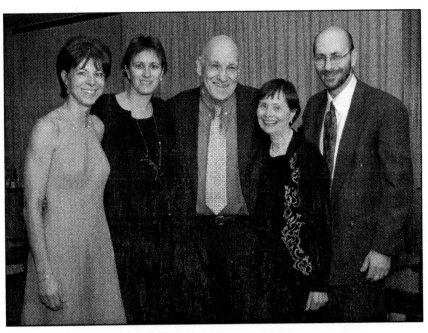

*Paul and me with our three children. From left
to right: Rachel, Rebecca, Paul, me and Joshua.
The picture was taken at our granddaughter
Danielle's Bat Mitzvah in March of 2007.*

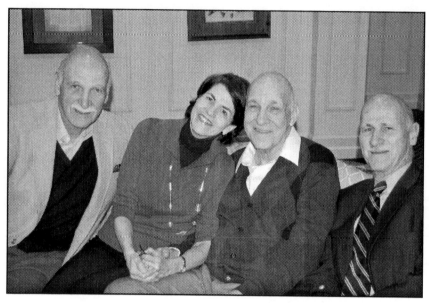

Paul's siblings joined us at our 50ᵗʰ anniversary celebration in January of 2008. From left to right: Mark, Irene, Paul and Carl.

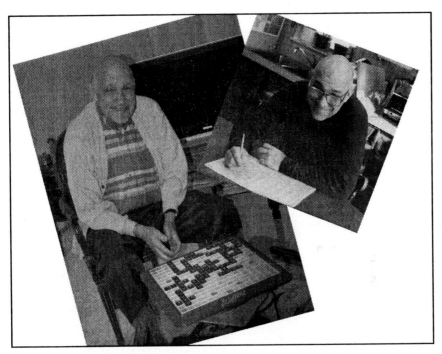

Although Paul always did crossword puzzles, he never played Scrabble until the Fall of 2010.

Chapter 3
TRANSITIONS

*H*aving to face the challenge of a devastating disease has enhanced my appreciation of life. I had to make a transition from anger and despair to acceptance. I needed to find meaning in my life and realize that nothing could have greater meaning than helping my life partner continue to have a good quality of life as long as possible.

I had to accept that my marriage as I had known it was over. How did I find that deeper love for Paul? I love my husband, and I've made our relationship my top priority. I am no longer busy raising children or working or having to find out who I am or having to keep proving myself. I can devote myself to Paul and his daily needs. This is what I have chosen to do.

I had to find sociability—communities that would accept both of us. Fortunately, we have The Glen with its stress-free living and built-in sociability. This retirement facility is not overwhelming for Paul to find his way around. Everyone knows everyone, and Paul feels very secure here.

I fully recognize that not everyone can move to a retirement community as we did. However, most areas have resources for Alzheimer's patients and support services for their spouses. For example, there are day-care centers, community volunteer programs, and assisted-living facilities.

My experience with Paul has made me a better person. I'm learning to love unconditionally. Learning to love— really love—someone else. When things are going well, it is easy to be loving. I'm learning how to love deeply.

I'm learning patience. I'm learning not to be defensive. Paul has no idea of my needs. At first it seemed as though he was becoming selfish and only thinking of himself. I've learned to accept that he has all he can do to think of himself. He can't be thoughtful of me.

I'm learning to change. He can't. And yet he is changing in the ways he shows me his love and puts his love into words of gratitude for all I do for him. These are thoughts that he never expressed as frequently in the past. Now he is so appreciative of everything that I do for him. Before his illness, he took so much for granted.

I'm learning to have an appreciation for the ordinary.

I'm learning not to have unrealistic expectations.

I'm learning that things change, and I have to keep up with the changes.

I'm learning I constantly need to plan ahead yet be flexible as plans change.

I'm learning to take care of myself. I recognize that it is important that my needs not be overlooked, and it is essential for me as the caregiver to have socialization. I stay in touch with family and friends and allow them to be supportive. I stay active and take care of myself. If I am not healthy, I cannot be an effective caregiver. Above all, I try to keep a positive attitude.

Living within the retirement community has provided me with the opportunity to become more self-aware and to be able to have the time for self-examination. I have facilitated a spiritual journey group in my home for fourteen years, and I continue to do so. I am a person who reflects and thinks things through. It is important that I not be just a caregiver. I don't want to be a martyr. I am not a martyr. I have a full life, and every day I think how fortunate I am to still have my husband.

Chapter 4

FACING CHALLENGES, ADAPTING, AND COPING WITH CHANGE

I have learned that the most difficult and yet most important basic concept for both me as the caregiver and for Paul is accepting the diagnosis of his Alzheimer's disease and all that it means. Denying it is all too often the reaction of both the patient and others. I vividly remember the day the doctor told me that I must take over. I accepted the challenge with trepidation. I knew that we were about to start a new journey together through uncharted territory.

From then on, I had to make decisions for both of us. I had to take over areas that were previously Paul's domain, such as our financial affairs. I was not prepared, and the responsibility seemed overwhelming at first. Our children helped me to become more confident in myself, and I realized that I was up to the challenge. I had to keep reminding myself that I have always loved a challenge, and that I could do it.

To channel my worrying, I concentrated on planning for the future. I took care of legal matters and downsized by selling our house and moving to the independent retirement residence The Glen at Hiland Meadows. Living there makes our lives as stress-free as possible. I made the decision to move because I wanted to use my energy helping us have a happy life together and not be saddled with the problems entailed in owning a home. This freed Paul of the frustrations he was feeling at not being able to keep up with the house maintenance and repairs. Moving also eliminated the arguments about my hiring people to do the jobs he had always done but could no longer handle.

An added benefit of downsizing our style of living while we were still able to make decisions about what we wanted to do with all our things—or "stuff," as Paul called it—was that we weren't leaving an overwhelming job for our children at a time of crisis. After we moved, each of our three children individually said to me, "Mom, do you realize you gave us the greatest gift of all when you sold your home and moved?" It gave great peace of mind to our children and relieved them of a great deal of worry.

A big help for me in meeting the challenge is being flexible and creative. For instance, as new people move into The Glen, I make sure Paul gets a chance to sit with them at dinner so that he can tell his stories and have a new audience.

I make use of positive reinforcement and conditioning.

I keep things structured. When it became apparent that traveling was no longer an option, we stopped traveling. It is important to join the world of the patient and not expect him to join our world and our expectations. I focus on attending the activities that Paul enjoys, like hockey games and concerts. Sports and music are two fields that he can still enjoy to the fullest, and sitting next to him at both is like old times before he had Alzheimer's. So it is a special feeling for me too. (By the way, I hate hockey!)

The major change is that I am now responsible for *everything!* I have had to learn on the job. Paul's short-term and long-term memory are both on a downward spiral, so I have to continually think of ways to help him. He knows I don't mind him using me as his memory. When we see someone, I'll always say the person's name so he can remember who it is. The same thing with a telephone call. Paul is no longer allowed to drive. I can still drive around town, but I don't drive on the highway anymore. I find it is too stressful. Also, I drive as little as possible at night. There are many activities that Paul no longer enjoys, like going to plays or belonging to a book club. So we don't do them anymore. He thrives on structure, and I keep things as structured as possible. I try to avoid leaving him home alone at night, but it is possible for me to go out for a short while during the day. It works best in the morning when he has a set routine. He goes to have coffee and chat with friends. He reads the paper and goes to the computer room to read online.

This is the way I cope. These are examples of what has worked for me. I hope my experience and the strategies shared in Chapter 6 of this book will help you find what works for you.

Chapter 5

How Our Faith Has Sustained Us

O ur faith has played an important part in sustaining us during these years. Paul and I are traditional Jews and belong to Congregation Shaaray Tefila, the conservative synagogue in Glens Falls. Our synagogue has always been an important part of our lives. In addition to satisfying our religious needs, the synagogue members are an important support group for us.

Each week we have a traditional Friday evening meal. I light the Sabbath candles; Paul sings the Kiddush, the prayer over the wine, and says the blessing over the bread. Although for the most part Paul has minimal memory now, he still remembers these prayers and melodies, and participating in these rituals each week gives him a special feeling, contributes to his self-esteem, and definitely lifts my spirits as well as his.

Judaism teaches us that we are God's partners, and

therefore we must do our part. I am grateful to be able to be Paul's caregiver, and I feel I'm doing holy work.

God has always played a central part in our lives, and now that Paul has Alzheimer's, I can't imagine what I would do if I didn't have God by my side.

Prayer plays an important part in our daily life. Each evening as we go to sleep, Paul thanks God for giving him me for his wife, and I thank God for bringing me Paul for my husband. We credit God for bringing us together and for our life together. Our spirituality helps carry us through life's challenges and gives meaning and purpose to our lives.

Daily, I thank God and am so grateful that we have as good a life as possible, considering the disease we're dealing with. I pray for good health so that I will be able to be there to care for Paul. I pray for patience, for guidance, for strength, and for me to have unconditional love for him despite the challenges of the disease. I pray that Paul will not experience physical pain.

I continue to attend Saturday morning services at the synagogue as well as the shorter Sunday morning services, but attending these services has become too much for Paul. He continues, however, to come to the once-a-month Friday evening service our synagogue holds at the retirement residence where we live. Paul still participates fully and remembers all the prayers and melodies.

Early each morning, I try to go for an hour's walk, and I find it to be a perfect time to meditate and have quiet conversations with God. These walks in nature and talks with God help me to keep being upbeat in my outlook.

I have a master's degree in spiritual direction, and for the past fourteen years I have been facilitating a spiritual journey group once a month in our apartment. Paul has always been a member of the group. The group has meant a great deal to both of us. Again, it provides a loving support group for us. We are surrounded by spiritual people with positive outlooks and positive vibes, and the group is very healing and supportive for all of us.

As you can see, religion and spirituality have played a major part in our coping with Alzheimer's.

Chapter 6

STRATEGIES

I've divided the strategies that have been useful for me into categories. Since every individual diagnosed with Alzheimer's is different, and so is every caregiver, no strategy will work for everyone. Use these as inspiration to find the strategies that work for you.

Unconditional Loving

- *I love Paul unconditionally.* He has the security of my love, even when the disease causes him to act in ways that are difficult to accept.
- *I hug and touch Paul as often as possible.* Even as his comprehension goes, he still feels and needs the reassurance of touch.

Simplifying Our Lives

- *I downsized our house and belongings.* We moved to The Glen, an independent-living facility with stress-free living.
- *I prioritized my time and energy.* Everything else moves to second place so that I have the necessary focus for Paul.

Social/Emotional

- *I tell everyone Paul has Alzheimer's disease.* Others become extra eyes for me.
- *I keep Paul content and involved as much as possible.* He is happiest when he is doing things he enjoys and doing things without feeling anxious.
- *I don't force Paul to do what he doesn't want to do.* I listen to him. If I treat him like a child, he acts rebellious.
- *I don't argue with Paul.* Rather, I distract and redirect him.
- *When Paul doesn't want to do something, such as shower, I accept his refusal.* I wait, and a short time later I ask him again.
- *I find ways that Paul can be helpful.* Performing chores around the house and contributing within the community helps boost his self-esteem.

- *I try hard to stay positive.* Paul feeds off my moods, so it is very important that my mood is good. I firmly believe that hope and positive energy can turn challenges into triumphs. So I look for the positive. When I find myself heading in a downward spiral, I consult a friend, a social worker, or a therapist. I know if I change the way I think, I will change the way I feel. There is no magic.

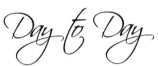

Day to Day

- *I keep things simple.* I speak in short sentences. I only ask him to do one thing at a time.
- *When I go out, I leave Paul a note telling him where I am.* I always leave the note in the same place, and I've trained him to do the same if he leaves the apartment.
- *I try not to over-schedule events.* Paul often requires a lot of extra sleep.
- *I encourage Paul to take care of himself.* This includes taking naps when he is tired.
- *I invite friends to come for lunch or dinner.* Paul still loves company.
- *I seek out and immerse myself and Paul in social activities.* I am willing to join Paul's world by participating in activities that interest him. I

53

change plans as I observe that activities are no longer pleasurable to him.

- *I use the interviewing technique to keep communication open.* See our "ings" interview in Chapter 2.
- *I remind myself that the behavior of Alzheimer's patients is similar to that of little children.* I try to guide and redirect Paul, while all the time ensuring that his dignity is maintained.

Dressing

- *I went through Paul's clothes in both his closet and bureau and made sure everything is easy to put on and matches.* This way, he can still pick out his own clothes and have a degree of independence.

Hygiene

- *As Paul became incontinent, I switched him to Depends.* It wasn't easy.

Medications

- *I have had to take charge of all of Paul's medications.* At first, Paul resented me when I tried to help him with his medicines. He insisted he could do it himself. It became apparent that he was not refilling his medicines on time and wasn't able to take care of them. His doctor had to help me convince him that I was on his team, and that he had to let me take over the meds. Paul would often help himself and confuse which day's pills to take. I had the challenge of getting him to stop helping himself and wait for me to hand him the pills. Paul has a lot of medicine that he has to take, and it is almost a full-time job ordering his medications and setting up the week's medicines.

Taking Messages

- *I do not expect Paul to take messages for me.* I tell callers that if I am not at home, they need to ask Paul to please hang up and tell him that they will call right back and leave me a message on our answering machine. Paul can't remember how to play back the messages, so that system works just fine. In the several years before he was diagnosed, Paul would take messages and then forget to tell me; people would be annoyed that I didn't call them back. Paul would think he could remember to tell me and wasn't aware that he no longer could rely on his memory. It didn't occur to him that he should write down the messages. I managed to program him to do that, but unfortunately, he would write the messages on little scraps of paper and leave the papers in miscellaneous spots. I might not find the message for days, if at all. I bought a pad to keep right next to the phone for him to write the messages on, but somehow, he never programmed himself to do it. Now we skip that altogether.

Inappropriate Behavior

- *I use positive reinforcement to condition appropriate behavior.* Very calmly and unemotionally, I repeat over and over the correct behavior in order to get him to change. I have to pick and choose the issues that are most important to me to assist him in changing his behavior. Paul has walked out in front of cars; he has gone up to speak to the rabbi while the rabbi is leading services. He hides his dirtied underwear in his closet. Once he gets something in his mind, this behavior becomes a pattern that he seems unable to change or to recognize as incorrect. The filters and processes for appropriate behavior are gone.

Maintaining Safety

- *I gave away our teakettle.* To replace it, I bought an electric teapot that shuts off automatically on its own.
- *I threw away our microwave oven.* Paul was confused in using the microwave and melted the sides. We were better off without one.
- *I replaced our toaster oven with a simple toaster Paul can manage.* I weaned him from using the stove and oven. It took time and patience, but it was well worth it.

Schedules — Daily and Weekly

- *I try to ensure that we maintain a daily routine.* Paul is most happy leading a very simple and structured life. Every day when he wakes up, he asks me what day it is and what we have to do that day. He sleeps late every day and then gets up and eats his breakfast. At times, he still showers himself and shaves. At other times, I have to remind him to shower. He prefers not to shave every day.
- *If we have an event later in the day, I suggest that he dress for that event from the start.* This saves him having to change later. Paul does not have a high

energy level, and once he is dressed, he does not like to change again. In fact, he gets very upset if he has to change his clothes during the day.

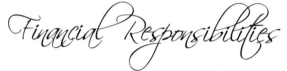

Financial Responsibilities

- *I had someone show me how to handle our household finances.* Paul had always been in charge of that. It was something he was good at, and I was thrilled to let him do it. I had no idea how to balance a checkbook or do the taxes. By the time it became apparent that he no longer could or should be in charge, he was beyond being able to teach me. I recognized when I needed help, and I was not embarrassed to ask for it.
- *I canceled Paul's credit cards.* We both used to have credit cards, but now they are all in my name, and I am the only one who writes checks and pays the monthly bills.
- *We worked with a lawyer to redefine the legal structure of our assets and redefine who could have access to them.* This became important when Paul was no longer able to handle financial matters.

Health Care
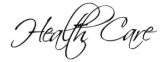

- *Many years ago, we both took out long-term care insurance.* We felt that in the event that nursing home care is required in the future, this insurance will be invaluable.
- *When the time comes, I plan to contact a hospice organization.* Regardless of the cause of illness or death, I strongly believe that hospice is invaluable in helping a person (and his family) through the process of dying.

Taking Care of Myself

- *I get some exercise every day.* As Paul's caregiver, I am extra aware of the importance of my well-being, so I'm learning to take better care of myself physically.
- *I eat healthy food.* I know I can't afford to get sick.
- *I try to get ample rest.* I know I need to work on this one.

Alzheimer's Association

- *The Alzheimer's Association has been a lifesaver for me.* With the Alzheimer's Association, I know that I am not alone. The Alzheimer's Association Helpline at 1-800-272-3900 is available twenty-four hours a day to answer any questions and give me emotional support. They can also be reached at www.alz.org.

Chapter 7
COMMENTS FROM OUR CHILDREN—REBECCA, RACHEL, AND JOSHUA

Traveling the Alzheimer's journey as Paul's children has involved and affected us, too. True, there's an inherent sadness that comes from being witness to the deterioration caused by the disease. Yet because of Mom's positive "ing" attitude and approach to being Dad's caregiver, and because of Dad's positive outlook on life, we, their children, have benefited from the journey in many "ing" ways.

Learning

One can't help but learn from Sunny and Paul. Mom's endless patience and her very strong communication skills have allowed us a window into what she's doing and why she's doing it. Dad has always taught us that one is never too old to learn, including his (still!) daily practice of using reference materials to complete crossword puzzles and to find answers to trivia questions that arise.

Growing

We've chosen to grow to meet the standard set by our parents. Never for a moment has their level of expectation for a high quality of life dropped—ever! And never will our efforts to support them both lessen.

Bonding

Never knowing how and when it will all end helps reframe family visits as golden opportunities. Minutes are valuable, hours are precious, and days are priceless. Each family Scrabble game (no keeping score!) and each meal shared around the dinner table are special experiences forever engraved in our memory.

Inspiring

The lessons learned from Sunny and Paul's journey with Alzheimer's have inspired each of us, as well as inspired us in our role as parents to our own children. Their nine grandchildren understand the situation completely, and rather than shy away from visits with Saba and Savta, they embrace their time together.

Humbling

Mom and Dad, in their setting of priorities, have helped us recognize that it's all about health, dignity, and quality of life. There's nothing more humbling than observing one's parents talk the talk and walk the walk.

Blessings

We thank Mom and Dad for all they have given us. We are truly blessed!

We are so proud to be the children of Sunny and Paul. Mom and Dad, there are no words to express our level of respect, gratitude and appreciation for you!